Hair Loss Cure

75 Natural Hair Growth Secrets and
Hair Loss Cure For Growing Long and
Fast Hair

HILDA McCRAY (PHD)

Limit of Liability

The information in this book is solely for informational
purposes, not as a medical instruction to replace the advice of
your physician or as a replacement for any treatment prescribed
by your physician. The author and publisher do not take
responsibility for any possible consequences from any treatment,
procedure, exercise, dietary modification, action or application of
medication which results from reading or following the
information contained in this book.

If you are ill or suspect that you have a medical problem, we
strongly encourage you to consult your medical, health, or other
competent professional before adopting any of the suggestions
in this book or drawing inferences from it.

This book and the author's opinions are solely for informational
and educational purposes. The author specifically disclaims all
responsibility for any liability, loss, or risk, personal or otherwise
which is incurred as a consequence, directly or indirectly, of the
use and application of any of the contents of this book.

ISBN-13: 978-1523953493

ISBN-10: 1523953497

DEDICATION

To all who desire to live life to the fullest!

TABLE OF CONTENT

INTRODUCTION

Are you starting to think more of natural hair lately? Or probably you have been natural for many years but sometimes you still feel like you don't have your routine down? Are you tired of store bought natural hair products that don't seem to give your hair enough of the moisture needed or define your curls?

This book has a list of homemade recipes that you can create yourself to use in your natural hair care routine. This book's recipes include homemade shampoos, conditioners, detanglers, growth potions and so on. Have u been having a lot of hair breakage or baldness...This book is the perfect answer

Natural homemade shampoo Recipes

Has it ever occurred to you to make your own shampoo? Yeah, probably not. With the hundreds of commercial shampoos that we have available in stores here and there, why bother making our own at home, right?

Well, I really think it is needful to stress the reasons why you should consider this option in the first place:

Benefits of homemade shampoo Recipes

Saving Money

Like with many other things, shampoo made at home is far cheaper than the commercial made shampoo. Most especially if you have a large family, making your own shampoo is ideal for you, and it would save you the extra cost.

Better for You

We don't know what all those chemicals are in your commercial conditioner and shampoo?

The FDA does not regulate what companies put in personal care products, which means most of us do not have any idea what the chemicals are or how they might be affecting us. The majority of large companies like Pantene, Suave and Aussie use chemicals that have been associated with the cause of cancer, allergies, immunotoxicity and so on.

Therefore making your shampoo yourself is safer for you and your family because you will be using natural ingredients.

Works Better

This is would be somehow highly subjective. Some people say that their homemade shampoo gives far better results than the commercial brands. Other people say they would rather buy commercial shampoo any day.

How well your shampoo works is going to be dependent on your choice of recipe, and as well as the type of your hair. But there is a great chance it will blow your store-bought shampoo out of the water…in a good way.

Better for the Environment

When you use natural shampoo what goes down the drain are natural ingredients. Commercial conditions and shampoos contain tons and tons of chemicals, which go right into our water system. So, natural shampoos are way better for the environment.

Better for Your Home

These natural ingredients are way better for your pipes. The harsh chemicals in the commercial brand conditions and shampoos can cause major damage to your pipelines over time, which will cost you big-time financially.

Homemade Shampoo Recipes

So how can you make your own shampoo? Fortunately there are tons of great homemade shampoo recipes out there. Here are two that I really like:

Castile Shampoo

Ingredients:

¼ cup of liquid Castile soap

¼ cup of water

½ tsp of oil (like grapeseed, olive oil or jojoba)

Direction:

Combine all three ingredients into glass bottle or a plastic.

NOTE

Some people are good with this combination; while some others says it leaves a film on their hair. Anyways, a lot depends on your type of hair and your type of water (hard water seems to leave more film).

Baking Soda Shampoo

Combine 3 cups of warm water with half cup of baking soda (this will produce enough for several washings). Store in a glass container or plastic.

When ready to use, shake and then apply to your scalp, scrubbing it in. After that, rinse with half cup of apple cider vinegar (or regular white vinegar for a lighter smell). You can also use 1 Tbsp of vinegar mixed with a cup of water for a lighter mixture. It is necessary that you have it in mind that there are as many natural shampoo recipes as there are people experimenting. You might need to play with proportions a little before you find a combination that works great for you.

NOTE:

It might take some time, probably 2 weeks or more for your hair to "settle in" to being washed with vinegar and baking soda. The reason is because right now, your hair has been daily stripped of natural oils because of commercial shampoo (and daily washing routines). When you go natural, your hair may start to feel greasy or thick as your body adjusts. Do not back out! It's also best to discipline yourself not to wash your hair every day, whether you are using natural shampoo or not. Washing every two days will help keep your hair and scalp healthy.

Basic Hair Shampoo

If you want normal hair, or as a base to add your own scents, you should use

Ingredients:

Foaming Bottles or Flip Cap Bottles to dispense

¼ cup of liquid Castile Soap (unscented or your favourite)

¼ cup of water (distilled)

½ tsp of grapeseed, jojoba or other light vegetable oil

Direction:

Combine together all the three ingredients. Store in any of the bottles above. Shake before use.

This mixture is not as thick as commercial brand shampoos – you will need to just tilt the bottle over your head.

The lather it makes is really impressive though!

Hair Stimulant Shampoo

To wake your senses and scalp up, try tea tree and peppermint oil! This one is my favorite, and the only one I use daily. It's so very refreshing!

Ingredients:

1/8 teaspoon o f tea tree essential oil

¼ cup of water (distilled)

1/8 teaspoon of peppermint essential oil

2 teaspoon of jojoba oil

¼ cup of liquid Castile Soap (unscented or your favorite)

Flip Cap Bottles or Foaming Bottles to dispense

Direction:

Combine all five ingredients, and then add ¼ cup of distilled water

Store in a bottle. Use as you would any commercial brand shampoo, rinse well.

Hair Quench Shampoo

For dry hair, try this:

Ingredients:

¼ cup of distilled water

¼ cup of aloe vera gel

¼ cup of liquid Castile Soap (your favorite scent)

¼ tsp of jojoba oil or avocado oil

1 tsp of glycerin

Flip Cap Bottles or Foaming Bottles to dispense

Directions:

Combine all five ingredients and then store in a bottle. Always shake well before using.

Hair Soothe Shampoo

Chamomile makes this 'poo a great and calming treat. Chamomile also comes with natural lightening properties, so you should combine this with lemon juice if you want to lighten your hair!

Ingredients:

1 ½ tbsps of glycerin

1 cup castille soap (use Lavender)

1 cup of water, distilled

6 chamomile tea bags

Flip Cap Bottles or Foaming Bottles to dispense

Directions:

Steep the teabags in a cup of boiled water for about twenty mins. Remove the tea bags and then discard. Add castille soap to the tea. Stir in the glycerin until it becomes well blended. Keep in a cool and dark place in a sealed bottle.

Hair De-Flake Shampoo

To correct a flaky scalp, this simple recipe is for you:

¼ cup of water, distilled

1 tbsp of apple cider vinegar

¼ cup of liquid Castile Soap

½ tsp of grapeseed, jojoba, or other light vegetable oil

6 finely ground cloves

3 tbsps of apple juice

Flip Cap Bottles or Foaming Bottles to dispense

Directions:

Combine all six ingredients in a blender or small grinder for thirty secs.

Wet your hair with warm water and shampoo the mixture into your hair well. Rinse with warm water.

Cover and put leftovers in a refrigerator. Discard after three days!

Hair Shine Shampoo

Lively and fragrant, to add shine to your hair, try this recipe

Ingredients:

2 tablespoons of rosemary, dried

¼ cup of water, distilled

¼ cup of liquid Castile Soap (use lemon)

¼ lemon essential oil

2 tablespoons sweet almond oil

Flip Cap Bottles or Foaming Bottles to dispense

Directions:

Boil distilled water; add rosemary and then steep until it is fragrant.

Strain the leaves and allow to cool. Combine all the ingredients and add to water and then stir to combine well. Store in a bottle. Use as you would use any commercial brand shampoo, rinse well.

Hair Fragrant Shampoo

The alluring smell of this luxurious shampoo is irresistible.

¼ cup liquid Castile Soap (your favorite)

¼ cup of water, distilled

10 drops of coconut fragrance oil

2 teaspoon of jojoba oil

10 drops of vanilla essential oil

Flip Cap Bottles or Foaming Bottles to dispense

Directions:

Combine all the ingredients together. Store in a bottle; and then use as you would any other shampoo, rinse well.

Try not to drink this shampoo. It smells super good. . .

Hair Dry Shampoo

Ingredients:

1 teaspoon of baking soda

¼ cup of oatmeal

1 teaspoon of lavender or other fragrant herb, crushed

Direction:

Using a mortar and pestle, or a small grinder, grind the ingredients.

Sprinkle enough mixture to cover all your hair, and rub in for 5 mins before brushing out

This could be produced in bulk and stored in a cool and dry place.

Natural hair conditioner recipe

Homemade natural hair conditioner is a far better way to target hair care treatments to your personal specific hair type - without synthetic additives or harmful chemicals.

Conditioning helps to protect your hair from stressors such as heat-styling, weather, poor diet, hormone fluctuations, etc. Conditioning also helps to re-moisturizes dry hair and also forms a layer of protection around the entire hair shaft, which helps to reduce breakage and split ends.

Best Carrier Oils for Your Hair Type

Use the information to help you customize your own natural hair conditioner recipe to your hair's particular needs. You also can blend these oils in any combination you like. Some people like a blend of coconut or shea and olive oil.

Normal Hair: Olive Oil, Jojoba Oil, Virgin Coconut Oil

Dry, Damaged or Frizzy Hair: Jojoba Oil, Shea Butter, Castor Oil, Olive Oil, Virgin Coconut Oil

Oily Hair: Jojoba Oil, Grapeseed Oil

Thinning Hair: Olive Oil, Castor Oil, Avocado Oil, Grapeseed Oil, Sweet Almond Oil

Dandruff: Castor Oil, Avocado Oil, Sesame Oil, Olive Oil, Virgin

Note: the avocado oil should only make up to 10 percent of the total oil hair care blend because it leaves a waxy residue that's very hard to rinse or wash out.

Basic Natural Hair Conditioner Recipe

Ingredients

½ cup of distilled Water or Herbal Infusion

1 tsp of Carrier Oil for your hair type (check table above)

1 tbsp of (8g) Emulsifying Wax

Essential Oil Blend for your hair type

½ teaspoon of Vitamin E (or 2 capsules)

1 tsp of Vegetable Glycerin

5 drops of Grapefruit Seed extract

Directions:

Stir to combine the oil, emulsifying wax and glycerin in the upper part of a double boiler, warming slowly over low heat until the wax becomes melted. Remove from the heat and pour in the Vitamin E.

In a microwave or in a separate pot on the stove, gently warm the water or herbal infusion just until it becomes lukewarm. It is important that you don't skip this step or your conditioner will separate later on.

Slowly pour in water or the herbal infusion into the oil mixture, stirring continuously with a wire whisk until the mixture becomes creamy and smooth. Let the mixture cool a little so that the essential oils do not evaporate too quickly when you add them. Don't worry if it doesn't thicken immediately - it thickens as it cools down to room temperature.

Stir in the grapefruit seed extract and the essential oils. Pour the natural hair conditioner into a clean, sterilized eight ounce (250ml) dark glass or PET plastic bottle and allow it to cool before covering.

Shake the bottle occasionally as the conditioner begins to cool down to prevent the ingredients from separating. Store in a cool and dark place.

Note: Some people have told me that this recipe makes their hair greasy. If that's also the case for you, use grapeseed oil, which is very light. You should also reduce the amount of carrier oil.

Herbs for Natural Hair Conditioner Recipes

Add an herbal infusion to your natural hair conditioner to enhance the color and also make your hair's appearance healthy of your hair.

Combine 1 tbsp of each of the appropriate herbs with ¼ cup of (60ml) distilled water in a small pot and bring to boiling on the stove. Remove pot from the stove and let steep for thirty mins to one hour.

Strain out the herbs and replace the water with your infusion in the basic conditioner recipe above.

Blonde Hair Peel	Chamomile, Dried Calendula, Lemon
Red Hair Bark	Hibiscus, Dried Calendula, Cinnamon
Dark Hair	Dried Rosemary, Black Tea, Cloves
Gray Hair	Rosemary, Dried Sage, Thyme

Note: The infusion for gray hair smells pretty "herbal", but people say it's really worth it because it brings back your original hair color if you use it daily.

Herbal care rinse

These are one of the best natural hair treatments anyone can use, and they are very easy to make. Using herbal hair rinse after natural hair conditioning reduces product buildup, balances the scalp's pH and boosts manageability and shine.

Herbal hair rinse also helps to heal irritation and inflammation caused by heat styling and chemical hair treatments. Especially very important for dandruff and oily hair.

How to make an herbal hair rinse:

Combine 2 cups (500ml) of distilled water with herbs (see table below) in a pot and bring to boiling, on a stove.

For Normal to Dry Hair: use three tbsps each of dried Chamomile and Lavender.

For Oily Hair, Thinning Hair or Dandruff: use three tbsps each of dried Peppermint and Rosemary.

Remove pot from heat and let steep for one hour. Strain out herbs and pour into a PET plastic bottle or large dark glass. Add two tbsps of Apple Cider Vinegar.

To use the herbal hair rinse, simply pour it over the hair after you have conditioned it, rub it gently into your scalp and then rinse.

Secret Recipe for Smoothing Frizzy Ends

Here's a quick one, a hair care trick for smoothing out frizzy, fly-away ends: Pour a very tiny, dime-sized amount of jojoba oil into the palm of your hand. Rub your palms together, and then smooth them over the fly away ends of your hair.

Do not rub over the hair near your scalp or you will weigh your hair down and it will look lank and greasy (this also happens if you use too much oil.)

NATURAL DEEPCONDITIONER RECIPES

Mayonnaise hair conditioner

Ingredients:

2 Eggs

Mayonnaise

Olive oil

Directions:

Beat 2 eggs and add to a cup of mayonnaise, mix in one table-scoop of olive oil and add to a mixing bowl. Combine all ingredients by shaking and apply thoroughly to dry and clean hair. Wear plastic cap and sit under a hood drier or use hand-held blow drier for twenty mins. Rinse the ingredients with cold water and shampoo as usual.

Tropical Delight hair conditioner

Ingredients:

1 Cup of coconut milk

2 tablespoon of Mango Butter/Oil

¼ Cup of Honey

Directions:

Combine ingredients. Warm slightly, and apply to clean damp hair. Wrap/cover for thirty minutes or more and then rinse.

Deep hair conditioner

Ingredients:

½ cup of any moisturizing conditioner as a base

1 tablespoon of honey (for shine)

½ of an avocado (emollient fats in avocado is great for your hair)

2 teaspoon of bjco (black jamaican castor oil)

1 tablespoon of mayonnaise (light protein)

2 teaspoon of coconut oil

(You can substitute the oils to fit your hairs likings!)

Directions:

Firstly blend/mix avocado with base condish, blend/mix until the avocado becomes smooth then add other ingredients and then leave on your hair for as long as you would like, under a shower cap

The Cinnamon Combo

It is great for giving your hair a shine and for hydrating your curls

Ingredients:

Cinnamon

Mayo

Honey

2 eggs

A little milk

Directions:

Combine all of the five ingredients together and heat a little bit, and then apply to hair for as long as you want, thirty minutes is okay

Warning: can be a little messy

Coconut yogurt conditioner

Ingredients:

1/2 cups of coconut milk

2 tbsp of olive oil

1 to 2 cups of yogurt

2 eggs

Directions:

Combine beaten eggs and oil. Add the coconut milk and enough yogurt to thicken conditioner. Mix all four ingredients, and apply conditioner in section, then put plastic bag over your hair and then leave on for thirty minutes or longer. Rinse out your hair

Coconut Rapture

This treatment is a real good and hot treatment to use on damaged hair or normal hair.

Ingredients:

1 teaspoon of calendula oil

1 tablespoon of coconut oil

Directions:

Combine ingredients in a bowl and stand over a pan of simmering water until it is melted. Mix together. Massage into the hair while it is still warm. Wrap a hot towel round the head and sit for at least five mins before rinsing with warm water.

Honey Shine

Deep treatment to condition the hair, it makes it soft and gives it shine.

Ingredients:

Some cond. (Aussie Moist)

1 1/3 cup of honey

1 cup of Coconut oil

1 inch of olive oil

3 tbs of Lemon Juice

Directions

In a big bowl, combine all THREE ingredients, EXCLUDING the oils. Poor oil in a bottle and leave the bottle in a hot cup of water for two mins. (Both Coconut oil and Olive oil). Firstly, put the mixed products on your washed hair and then pour the oil on your hair also. Put a plastic cap on and wash out after thirty minutes or stay thirty minutes under the dryer if you want.

Deep conditioning mask with aloe vera

It can be used for any hair type.

Ingredients:

Aloe Vera (gel or fresh gel from leafs)

Green Tea

Coconut oil

Rosemary

Fresh ginger

Any Essential oil

Directions

Heat hot water in a stove, and then add the green tea, bring to boiling for about two mins; add coconut oil, rosemary, fresh ginger and aloe vera. Bring to a boil for five mins and then remove from the heat. Let it cool down and filter it with a tea strainer or anything you might prefer. Add two/three drops of any essential oil you may like. If coconut doesn't suit your kind of hair, you can replace it with some other oil. This is just a basic recipe, you can very well leave ingredients out or add or subtracts, that works perfectly fine. Adding an egg to the mixture would also be very good for the hair. Apply this to your scalp and continue to the ends, make sure to cover the ends properly because they are dry. You can apply it with a clean hair coloring brush, simply with your hands or a spray bottle. You can leave it in the hair for as long as you may want to, but at least for one hour, and it's good to steam your hair while the mask is in the hair. This mask would work well for any kind of hair, it is great for deep conditioning and it gives the hair some shine and leaves it soft.

HAIR DETANGLER RECIPES

Aloe Vera Detangler & Leave-In

This mix can be used as a leave-in and also a detangler. It can be used to detangle hair before shampooing or conditioner washing.

Ingredients

Aloe Vera juice

Grapeseed oil or essential oil

Directions:

Put one part grapeseed oil and three parts of aloe vera juice into a spray bottle and shake up. Section your hair into at least four sections. Then spray a section liberally with the mixture until it becomes drenched, smoothing it in with your hands to ensure that each of strand is well coated. Detangle the section with either a wide toothed comb or your fingers. Repeat on each of the remaining three sections. Wash and style your hair as usual. OR possibly you like to detangle while your hair is coated in conditioner, follow steps one to five steps after shampooing and apply the conditioner on top of the aloevera mix. Detangle your hair as usual.

Juicy Curly Magic

Ingredients:

6 ½ -7 ounces of Aloe Vera Juice

8 ounce Spray Bottle

Essential Oils (optional)

1 tablespoon of Jojoba Oil

1 tablespoon of Avocado Oil

Directions

Fill Spray Bottle with the aloe vera juice and measure in the oils. Keep in a refrigerator. Shake mixture well before use as the oils have a tendency to clump together from refrigeration. This mixture will have a natural aloe vera smell, which is good. But to mask the scent due to a dislike, or for a nice hair fragrance add in a couple drops of your favorite essential oil. You can use Sweet Orange, Vanilla or Lemon.

NATURAL HAIR BUTTER RECIPES

Whipped Shea butter

Ingredients

Shea butter, Olive oil, Almond oil, Jamaican black castor oil, tee tree oil, Coconut oil, Vitamin E oil.

Directions

Heat water up until it steams. Put shea butter into a small bowl to fit in the bowl of hot water. Allow the shea butter to melt, add one tbsp of olive oil, one tbsp of coconut oil, two tsp of almond oil, one tsp of Jamacian black castor oil, tee tree oil and vitamin e oil. Combine together, whisk using an egg beater.

All over Butter

Ingredients

10 drops of your favorite essential oil

8 ounce of unrefined organic Shea Butter

1 tablespoon of 100 percent Jojoba oil

Directions

Combine jojoba oil and the shea butter by mixing it together in a bowl with a hand mixer. When the jojoba and shea butter have blended together, add ten drops of the favorite essential oil of your choice. Once all the ingredients become mixed together, place the mixture into a storage container with a cover. This can be used as a body butter to be used after having a shower or as a sealant for your curls and kinks.

Whipped shea butter moisterizer

Ingredients

Oil (any one of these: flax seed oil, grape seed oil, olive oil, vegei oil, jojoba oil, fish oil.

Unrefined or Raw shea butter

Coconut oil, tee tree oil or castor oil.)

Directions:

Take as much ounces of Shea butter that you want and put it in a deep enough bowl for mixing. Combine in the oils, 1 tsp of each (if you have above six oils), a tbsp of each (if you have under six oils).

Now mix to combine, an electric mixer makes mixing easier, if you have one; or you can hand mix with a big wooden spoon.

Pumpkin Seed Butter Mask

Ingredients:

2 tablespoons of Dastony 100% Organic Sprouted Pumpkin Seed Butter

2 tablespoons of Sunny Isle Jamaican Black Castor Oil Extra Dark

2 tablespoon of GPB Glycogen Protein Balancing Conditioner

Directions:

Combine equal parts of the Castor Oil, Pumpkin Seed butter and conditioner. Apply to slightly damp or dry hair. You might need to add more conditioner for easier application...this mixture DOESN'T provide slip, it is a mask, so it just needs to get worked on the strands and into the hair. Cover hair with a plastic shower cap for at least an hour. By this time the mask will be dry stiff. Rinse and cleanse. Some people use it as a pre treatment to their wash day regimen, but it is also used as a deep conditioner as well! (It's necessary to still rinse out with a favorite conditioner if you use as a dc, for detangling and to make sure all the product has been removed)

Exotic Moisture Hair Cream

Ingredients

Unrefined mango, illipe butter and Tamanu oil, organic Aloe Vera Juice, Shea butter, 100 percent unrefined coconut oil, rosehip seed oil, organic aloe Vera gel, extra virgin olive oil, vitamin E oil and tea tree oil

Directions

Melt two heaping tbsps of unrefined mango, illipe and Shea butter in a microwave to a liquid, and then add three tbsps of each oil. Add approx. six to nine drops of tea tree oil and three to six drops of unrefined vitamin E oil. Mix in three tbsps of Aloe Vera juice and eight tbsps of aloe

Vera gel. Get a hand mixer and a plastic bowl. Mix until it becomes a creamy texture. Store in a refrigerator after use. It's can also be used as a body cream, isn't that lovely?

Cacao Hair Mask

Ingredients

1 teaspoon of pure cocoa powder

2 tablespoons of melted cocoa butter

1 tablespoons of extra virgin olive oil

2 tablespoons of vegetable shortening

Directions

Combine all ingredients together; Apply to ends and edges of your hair. Pin your hair up and out of the way and allow the mask to soak in for fifteen to thirty minutes.

Follow with your shampoo and conditioning regimen.

M's Hair Balm

Ingredients

1/8 cup of Saffron Oil

1 ounce or 1 stick of Coco Butter

3 Tablespoons of Shea Butter

1/8 - ¼ cup of Olive Oil

3 Tablespoons of Coconut oil

Directions:

Melt the Shea butter, Coconut and Coco Butter together in a container (the best container would be a tub of products that have cleaned out) until it becomes completely liquid. Stir in the Saffron and Olive oil until the container is full. Cover and place in a fridge for it to cool.

At room temp it should be a semi solid that melts easily in the hands when you want for use.

Enjoy the use of this product. Some people often use this after the leave in conditioner before the use of curl defining product to moisturize the scalp and tips of the hair. The result has been significantly softer (still much defined) curls since they start to use this.

NATURAL HAIR OIL RECIPES

Apricot Hair oil

This oil is good for twist and braids.

Ingredients

1oz. of Coconut Oil

2 oz. of Apricot oil

1 oz. of Jojoba Oil

1 tbsp of each Avocado Oil and Safflower Oil.

Directions:

Combine all four ingredients; apply to hair by massaging a generous amount in hair as needed for dry hair.

DIY Hair Oil using Jamaica Black Castor Oil

Ingredients

Empty bottle (2 ounce) with cap

Jamaica Black Castor Oil

Essential oil for fragrance (optional)

Grapeseed Oil

Droppers

Directions

Firstly, fill a bottle halfway with Jamaica Black Castor Oil (if necessary, use a dropper), using another dropper (different), add 2 tbsps of Grapeseed Oil. Tightly close the bottle cap, shake and your oil is ready to use.

Olive and coconut hair oil

Ingredients

4 ounce of coconut oil

3 ounce of olive oil

Directions

Mix the ingredients together, Put it in a bottle and apply every other day

1 inch in 1 week hair growth oil

Ingredients

Your favorite oil: extra virgin or coconut olive

(Any scalp oil of your choice)

Directions

Warm about two to three tablespoons of your favorite scalp oil and massage over your scalp and hair. Bend over so that your head is completely downwards. Note: You should be looking underneath the seat you are sitting on. This is known as inversion. It reverses the blood flow to the scalp to get hair growing. Invert for five minutes while giving a scalp massage. Do the oil and inversion for Seven days and you should see good results!

WARNING: if you are pregnant or unhealthy do not invert please. If you feel dizzy or light headed when inverting, DON'T DO IT.

Olive Oil Hair Mask

Ingredients

2 eggs

5 tbsps of olive oil

Directions

Combine eggs with olive oil. Apply thoroughly, massaging in to the hair. Wrap head with a shower cap or a plastic wrap. After 15 mins rinse well.

Herbal Oil Hair Treatment

Ingredients:

1 cup organic carrier oil

3-5 tbsps of herbs of your choice

Tightly closed container and jar

Directions:

Place about three to five tbsps of herbs in a glass jar. Cover with one cup organic carrier oil. Steep this mixture in a tightly closed jar for 2 weeks. On a daily basis, shake the jar. Once it is infused, strain out the herbs.

If you don't want to wait for two weeks, you can speed up infusion by gently warming the mixture on a stove at a very low heat for about fifteen too twenty mins and then steep overnight. It can be refrigerated for up to six months. Infused Oil

Egg & Olive Oil Hair Mask

Ingredients:

4 tablespoons of olive oil

2 whole eggs

Directions:

Combine olive oil and eggs. Smooth through the hair. Wrap your head with plastic wrap, and leave in your hair for ten mins. And then rinse well.

Hair Growth Hot Oil Treatment

Ingredients

3 drops of essential oil of thyme

1/8 cup of jojoba oil

3 drops of essential oil of lavender

3 drops of essential oil of rosemary

1/8 cup of grapeseed oil

3 drops of essential oil of cedarwood

Directions:

Combine all the ingredients. Then apply at night, to scalp in thinning areas. Do not rinse it out till morning.

Oil Blend for Hair Growth

Ingredients

3 drops cedarwood essential oil

1/8 cup jojoba oil

3 drops lemon essential oil

1/8 cup grapeseed oil

3 drops rosemary essential oil

3 drops lavender essential oil

3 drops thyme essential oil

Directions:

Combine all ingredients together. Apply several drops of the mixture to areas where you are experiencing hair loss each night, massaging gently into your scalp for three to five mins. Store oil in a tightly covered container and keep away from light and heat. If you are pregnant, avoid rosemary essential oil.

Lush Mane Oil

Ingredients

1 teaspoon of neem oil (optional)

1 tablespoon of castor oil

1 tablespoon of organic argan oil

Few of drops essential oils (optional)

1 tablespoon of coconut oil

1 tablespoon of olive oil

1 tablespoon of broccoli seed oil

Directions:

Before you start, make certain that your hair is dry and clean. Combine all the oils and warm them up if like it warmed. Pour some of the mixture and massage onto your scalp, adding more oil as you need. Spread the rest of the oil throughout the hair evenly (you may tweak the ingredients to make more). Use a shower cap and wear overnight. By morning, use a mild clarifying shampoo, to wash the oil out. Condition the hair and style as usual.

Use this treatment once in a week, and enjoy the results!

All natural Hot Oil treatment

Ingredients

Castor Oil

Olive Oil

Directions:

Mix olive oil and castor oil. Heat up and apply to your hair and scalp from the tips to root. It can also be used before washing the hair. Leave on hair for an hour or more if you want.

Valerie's Hairdrenalin Potion

Ingredients

½ large bottle of Cayenne Pepper

45 cut tea bags

2-4 drops onion seed oil

30 Biotin pills (blended or powder form)

2:1 ratio of onion seed oil to garlic seed oil (very dry)

1-2 drop garlic seed oil

Directions:

Combine all the ingredients together except the onion and garlic oil or powder, save it for the end. Infuse the mixture in an oven for about five hours. Remove from oven, set aside to cool down and stir occasionally. Once it is cooled, pour the oil into a container with a cheesecloth to separate the tea from the oil. Add the garlic and onion oil (or powder)

Keep out of the sunlight.

NATURAL HAIR GROWTH PORTIONS

Mustard Mask for Hair Growth

Ingredients

2 tablespoons of olive oil

2 tablespoons of ground mustard powder

1 egg yolk

2 teaspoons of sugar

2 tablespoons of hot water

Directions:

Combine water with mustard, add yolk, oil and sugar and combine very well. Part the hair into sections and put mix on the scalp. Do not put it on your hair ends. After you have applied to your hair, put on a plastic shower cap and on the top of it something warm to keep the heat in. It will heat up very quickly but that is very normal. It might start burning, but it's a good burn. But if you feel it's like an allergic reaction burn or so uncomfortable that you cannot take it, wash it out. Sit for a minimum of fifteen mins (maximum up to one hour).

After a minimum of fifteen mins, rinse the mask with warm water until the water runs and clear and then use you can use your favorite shampoo. It is advised that the mask should be done at least twice in a week for at least one or two months depending how slowly your hair grows.

1 inch in 1 week hair growth oil

Ingredients

Your favorite oil: extra virgin or coconut olive

(Any scalp oil of your choice)

Directions

Warm about two to three tablespoons of your favorite scalp oil and massage over your scalp and hair. Bend over so that your head is completely downwards. Note: You should be looking underneath the seat you are sitting on. This is known as inversion. It reverses the blood flow to the scalp to get hair growing. Invert for five minutes while giving a scalp massage. Do the oil and inversion for Seven days and you should see good results!

WARNING: if you are pregnant or unhealthy do not invert please. If you feel dizzy or light headed when inverting, DON'T DO IT.

Natural Growth Stimulating Conditioner

Ingredients:

¼ cup of plain natural yogurt

1 egg

1 teaspoon of fresh lemon juice

8 to 10 drops of eucalyptus oil (or olive oil, or rosemary oil, or rosemary/olive oil and canola oil)

Directions:

Process all the ingredients together in a blender. Massage onto and scalp hair and leave for a minimum of twenty to thirty mins before washing out.

Essential Growth Oil

Ingredients

½ teaspoon of jojoba oil

3 drops of lavender

2 drops of rosemary

2 drops of thyme

4 teaspoon of Grape seed oil (carrier oil)

Direction:

Combine all five ingredients well and then massage into the scalp for 2 mins. To increase absorption, wrap a warm towel around your head. With a mild shampoo, wash the hair after an hour. Make this a daily routine for at least 7 months.

Use a spray or an applicator bottle to apply to scalp as you need (on a daily basis).

The Healthy Hair Grow mixture

Ingredients

2 avacados

1 or 2 bananas (depending on the length of your hair)

2 teaspoons of shea butter

2 to 3 drops of tea tree oil

1 drop of eucalyptus oil

Directions:

You can mix or blend all ingredients together and put in a bowl. Wait until you conclude shampooing and conditioning your hair, then you distribute it evenly into your hair. Massage effectively into your hair and scalp. Then comb your hair with a wide tooth comb and leave in for five to ten mins.

Rinse your hair out thoroughly.

Coconut and Honey Cooling Hair Mask

Ingredients:

Castor oil

Avocado oil

Peppermint essential oil

Olive oil

Raw honey

Shea Moisture Raw Shea Butter Deep Treatment Masque

Organic Coconut Milk

Directions:

Mix in the castor, honey, olive and avocado oils together. Stir until it becomes smooth. Mix the Shea moisture deep conditioning mask and coconut milk together. Stir until it becomes smooth.

Add the oil and honey mix to the coconut milk and Shea moisture mix stir until it becomes smooth. The mixture should be creamy and thick.

If you want additional scalp stimulation add ten to twenty drops of peppermint essential oil drops to the final mixture. Apply the mix to a clean and freshly washed hair. Leave on for a minimum of thirty minutes. Rinse with cool water.

NATURAL HAIR GEL RECIPES

Aloe and Egg White Hair Gel

Ingredients

Whites from 3 eggs

1-2 Tablespoons of Vegetable Glycerin

2/3 cup aloe Vera gel

5-8 drops essential oil of choice (I use orange and some vanilla extract for a havenly smell.

1/8 cup of water

Directions

Combine all ingredients together in a small blender and blend for twenty seconds. Pour into a small sealable container. Put in a fridge until you are ready to use.

Vegan Chamomile & Mint styling gel

Ingredients

1 tablespoon of lemon juice

1/2 teaspoon of xanthan gum powder

1 tablespoon or 2 teabags of chamomile

1 cup water

½ tablespoon or 1 teabag of mint

1/3 cup aloe vera juice (the edible kind, can be substituted with water but this weakens the hold)

1 teaspoon maple syrup

Directions:

Boil the water and add the mint and chamomile, like you would brew regular tea. Let it steep until the liquid has become cooled to room temperature. Strain the herbal tea. Whisk all the ingredients together and let it rest for a moment. The xanthan gum will thicken slowly. You can also mix in a blender if you feel it's easier than whisking. You can then adjust the thickness to your liking easily. Add a tiny bit more xanthan gum powder if you find it is not as thick, on the other hand add water if it becomes too thick.

Aloe Pectin Hair Jelly

Ingredients:

1 cup of Aloe Vera juice

1 (1.59ounce) packet of instant fruit pectin

¼ teaspoons of Honey

¼ teaspoons of Agave Nectar

2 teaspoon of EVOO

1 teaspoon of Sweet Almond Oil

Directions:

Slowly add pectin into a bowl; note it should be slowly to avoid clumps, add aloe Vera juice to it, stirring from time to time. Add agave nectar, honey, evoo and sweet almond oil and mixed together. You can add essential oils for fragrance. Then put the already made gel in a squeeze/pump bottle or bowl with lid. Store in a refrigerator

Thick n' dreamy moisturizing styling cream

Ingredients

6 tbsps of your favorite moisturizing conditioner

12 tbsps of aloe vera gel

2 pinches cinnamon

½ tsp of your favorite oil (you can use evoo)

2 tsps of blue agave nectar

Your favorite essential oils (you can use tea tree and jasmine)

Directions:

Measure to combine all ingredients, using your discretion to get desired consistency. Whip or mix thoroughly

The final result or consistency is lighter than a gel but slightly thicker than the average styling cream; this makes it difficult to get into some containers. You can store in a glass jar).

Shake-n-go Natural Curls

Ingredients

1 jar or tube of Non-Flaking Gel or Aloe

1 tablespoon avocado oil, coconut oil, olive oil, mango butter, jojoba oil

2 tablespoons of pure shea butter,

Directions

Mix to combine, and then apply to hair that's wet and massage cream into your hair and scalp using your fingers to comb your hair in and form definition, shake hair and go.

Spritz All in one Styling Spray

Ingredients

2 teaspoons of Salt (epsom works perfectly)

1 cup hot water

1/3 cup gel

1 tablespoon of Oil (Jojoba, Olive, etc)

2 tablespoons of Conditioner

Directions

Combine ingredients in, put in spray bottle, shake very well, and keep in a refrigerator. Spray on your wet hair to style or dry hair to refresh/revive hair mid-day.

In a hot weather, you should leave out the oil from the ingredients and add a bit of honey and/or aloe as substitute. Effectiveness of this product can vary depending on brands of product used. Enjoy while experimenting.

1 inch in 1 week hair growth oil

Ingredients

Your favorite oil: extra virgin or coconut olive

(Any scalp oil of your choice)

Directions

Warm about two to three tablespoons of your favorite scalp oil and massage over your scalp and hair. Bend over so that your head is completely downwards. Note: You should be looking underneath the seat you are sitting on.

This is known as inversion. It reverses the blood flow to the scalp to get hair growing. Invert for five minutes while giving a scalp massage. Do the oil and inversion for Seven days and you should see good results!

WARNING: if you are pregnant or unhealthy do not invert please. If you feel dizzy or light headed when inverting, DON'T DO IT.

Mustard Mask for Hair Growth

Ingredients

2 tablespoons of olive oil

2 tablespoons of ground mustard powder

1 egg yolk

2 teaspoons of sugar

2 tablespoons of hot water

Directions:

Combine water with mustard, add yolk, oil and sugar and combine very well. Part the hair into sections and put mix on the scalp. Do not put it on your hair ends. After you have applied to your hair, put on a plastic shower cap and on the top of it something warm to keep the heat in. It will heat up very quickly but that is very normal. It might start burning, but it's a good burn. But if you feel it's like an allergic reaction burn or so uncomfortable that you cannot take it, wash it out. Sit for a minimum of fifteen mins (maximum up to one hour).

After a minimum of fifteen mins, rinse the mask with warm water until the water runs and clear and then use you can use your favorite shampoo. It is advised that the mask should be done at least twice in a week for at least one or two months depending how slowly your hair grows.

Essential Growth Oil

Ingredients

½ teaspoon of jojoba oil

3 drops of lavender

2 drops of rosemary

2 drops of thyme

4 teaspoon of Grape seed oil (carrier oil)

Direction:

Combine all five ingredients well and then massage into the scalp for 2 mins. To increase absorption, wrap a warm towel around your head. With a mild shampoo, wash the hair after an hour. Make this a daily routine for at least 7 months.

Use a spray or an applicator bottle to apply to scalp as you need (on a daily basis).

The Healthy Hair Growth mixture

Ingredients

2 avacados

1 or 2 bananas (depending on the length of your hair)

2 teaspoons of shea butter

2 to 3 drops of tea tree oil

1 drop of eucalyptus oil

Directions:

You can mix or blend all ingredients together and put in a bowl. Wait until you conclude shampooing and conditioning your hair, then you distribute it evenly into your hair. Massage effectively into your hair and scalp. Then comb your hair with a wide tooth comb and leave in for five to ten mins.

Rinse your hair out thoroughly.

Hair Growth Hot Oil Treatment

Ingredients such as rosemary helps to stimulate growth of hair, while it clears away of impurities and nourishing the scalp.

Ingredients

3 drops of essential oil of lavender

1/8 cup of grapeseed oil

3 drops of essential oil of rosemary

3 drops of essential oil of cedarwood

1/8 cup of jojoba oil

3 drops of essential oil of thyme

Directions

Combine all six ingredients together and then apply at night before sleeping, to your scalp in the thinning areas. Don't rinse out until it is morning.

Natural Growth Stimulating Conditioner

Ingredients:

¼ cup of plain natural yogurt

1 egg

1 teaspoon of fresh lemon juice

8 to 10 drops of eucalyptus oil (or olive oil, or rosemary oil, or rosemary/olive oil and canola oil)

Directions:

Process all the ingredients together in a blender. Massage onto and scalp hair and leave for a minimum of twenty to thirty mins before washing out.

Oil Blend for Hair Growth

Although there is no much guarantee that this blend will stimulate growth, many people have reported that they noticed a difference in the length of their hair

Ingredients

1/8 cup jojoba oil

3 drops thyme essential oil

3 drops lemon essential oil

3 drops cedarwood essential oil

3 drops rosemary essential oil

3 drops lavender essential oil

1/8 cup grapeseed oil

Directions

Combine all seven ingredients together in a small bowl, and place in a bottle. Shake well and then apply several drops of the mixture to your scalp and other areas of hair loss each night, massaging gently into your scalp for three to five mins. Store the oil tightly covered and kept away from heat and light.

NOTE: A pregnant woman should avoid rosemary essential oil.

ACV Growth Rinse

This hair growth portion is perfect as a final rinse and helps to promote and enhance hair growth. Rosemary has been used for several hundreds of years as a scalp stimulator.

Ingredients:

2 Tablespoons of Rosemary Dried Leaf

1 cup of Apple Cider Vinegar

1 cup of water

Directions

Place the rosemary in vinegar. Microwave the mixture for thirty seconds. Spoon the leaves that remained from the vinegar on the side of the jar. Strain the vinegar with the smallest available strainer you can lay your hands on (I recommend cut up pantyhose) and then add water. Apply as a final rinse.

Coconut and Honey Cooling Hair Mask

Ingredients:

Castor oil

Avocado oil

Peppermint essential oil

Olive oil

Raw honey

Shea Moisture Raw Shea Butter Deep Treatment Masque

Organic Coconut Milk

Directions:

Mix in the castor, honey, olive and avocado oils together. Stir until it becomes smooth. Mix the Shea moisture deep conditioning mask and coconut milk together. Stir until it becomes smooth.

Add the oil and honey mix to the coconut milk and Shea moisture mix stir until it becomes smooth. The mixture should be creamy and thick.

If you want additional scalp stimulation add ten to twenty drops of peppermint essential oil drops to the final mixture. Apply the mix to a clean and freshly washed hair. Leave on for a minimum of thirty minutes. Rinse with cool water.

Coconut Milk & Oil Recipe for Shiny Waves

This conditioning mixture is good when you want your curls moisturized. It works perfectly on normal, dry or oily hair. It strengthens your hair and adds shine to it, so it's also good for correcting hair loss and enhancing hair growth.

Ingredients

1 tablespoon of your favorite hair conditioner (you can use Senscience's Inner

Restore Intensif masque... but your choice matters)

1 tablespoon of Cane molasses

3 tablespoon of Coconut milk (or add to taste)

1 tablespoon of Coconut Oil

1 tablespoon of Honey

1 tablespoon of Rosemary infused Olive oil (or just plain olive oil)

Directions:

Combine ingredients manually in a small bowl or on a mixer, whatever works for you. Divide your hair into 4 sections and apply mixture from roots of your hair to the hair ends on every section, massaging the hair portion as you apply the mixture.

Do not rinse out immediately, you should leave it on for a minimum of an hour or for as long as you wish. Apply it on your hair that is pre-shampooed or second or third day hair (make sure it's still very clean).

NOTE: You can substitute the olive oil for any other oil of your choice.

Caribbean Smoothie

This hair growth portion leaves your hair silky, smooth and soft and also strong and very healthy. It also helps with rapid hair growth!

Ingredients

NOTE: ingredients can be tweaked, depending on the length of hair.

½ avocado (ripe)

½ cup of Coconut milk

½ banana (ripe)

1 tablespoon of Castor oil

2 tablespoon of Rosemary

1 teaspoon of Cayenne Pepper

Directions:

Combine all six ingredients in a blender, and process until it becomes smooth. Then apply the mixture from the ends of your hair to the roots and massage it in. Leave in for fifteen minutes to one hour. Rinse out completely with warm water.

Protein Humectant Deep Conditioner

This wonderful hair growth portion, PHDC retains moisture and it also adds protein to the hair –those are 2 key factors in hair growth and strength!

Ingredients

5 drops peppermint oil

1/4C extra virgin olive oil

1 egg

1/8C honey

1 avocado

1 teaspoon of biotin powder

Directions:

Combine all six ingredients together until it has a consistency that looks batter-like. Apply a generous amount to dry or damp hair. Cover your hair with a plastic cap or towel or both towel and plastic cap and/or sit under a dryer. Let the conditioner sit for thirty mins to one hour. Rinse with cool water.

Aloe Vera and Oil Shampoo

This hair growth is anti-fungal, anti-bacterial and hair growth promoting

Ingredients:

Water

Aloe Vera gel (better if it's fresh)

essential oils (rosemary, olive, castor, canola....)

Directions:

Blend some of the aloe Vera gel and ¼ or ½ of a cup of water and an essential oil of your choice (olive or rosemary or castor oil). Process in a blender till it becomes smooth and then pour into a container

Mayo Deep Treatment

This treatment is full of moisturizing agents, protein and more. You should use this treatment as a deep conditioning treatment to quench the thirst in your curls! it also helps to promote the growth of hair.

Ingredients:

3 tablespoons Honey

4 drops of Peppermint EO

4 tablespoons of Real Mayo

EVOO

1 Egg

EVCO

4 drops of Rosemary EO

Directions

Combine all seven ingredients together, mix thoroughly.
And then apply to your hair after shampooing. Leave on
for a minimum of one hour. Rinse well with cool water.

Homemade Leave-in Conditioner

This recipe promotes hair growth, prevents hair loss, prevents dandruff, cleanses the hair and scalp, prevents dry and itchy scalp, among many other things it does.

Ingredients:

10 small squirts of Lime Juice (naturally cleanses the hair and scalp, removes hair odors, prevents dandruff)

½ cup of Aloe Juice and gel (great for hair loss, a natural conditioner, great for dry and itchy scalps)

1 cup purified water

Milk/Water from 1 coconut

1 tablespoon of melted Shea butter, vitamin E (decreases sun damage, promotes growth, antioxidant)

1tablespoon of melted Coconut Oil

1 teaspoon of Olive oil (prevents dandruff and moisturizes)

½ teaspoon of Thyme oil (gives natural shine, promotes healthy scalp and prevents hair loss)

1 teaspoon of Rosemary oil (prevents hair loss, promotes growth, moisturizes and prevents dandruff)

Directions:

Combine all ingredients together and blend until it becomes smooth. When it is finely blended, transfer into a spray bottle.

Protein Deep Conditioner with Castor Oil

I started using this recipe about two months ago and I really love it for my hair. It is a simple recipe that consists of the usual mayonnaise and egg ingredients; but I also learnt to tweak and incorporate more ingredients

Ingredients:

1 tbsp of mayonnaise

1 egg

1 tsp of cold pressed castor oil

1-2 tsps of olive oil

1 drop of vitamin E oil

1 tbsp of rinse out conditioner (if desired, just in case may want some extra moisture)

NOTE: You can decide to double the ingredients if you have a lot of hair length. In the making of this recipe, the amount of ingredients that was used is for a twelve inches long hair or lesser.

Directions:

Combine all ingredients well in an empty bowl until it becomes well blended.

Divide your hair into sections for better distribution and apply to washed hair. Work the conditioner into each separate section.

Make sure you saturate your hair well!

Cover your hair with a plastic cap and leave on for twenty to thirty mins (You can also choose to sit under a dryer or heated cap for half the time); Rinse and wash out using your regular rinse out conditioner!

NOTE: you can use any essential oil that catches your fancy to trap the moisture. Feel the softness of your hair. Hope you like it!

Ayurvedic mask

This is a protein ayurvedic mud mask that is certain to send your curls poppin. This recipe certainly strengthens any coil, curl or kink back into shape and provides long lasting elasticity. The Brahmi in the ingredients promotes growth of hair

Ingredients:

Aloe vera juice or Coconut Milk

Ayurvedic henna mixture which includes Brahmi, hibiscus powder, shikakai, aloe vera, amla, bhringraj, neem, and jatamansi powders. You can use Nupur henna gotten from most local indian stores which includes all this in one package.

Your favorite moisture rinse out conditioner

One large egg

Coconut oil

Agave nectar or Honey

Directions

It depends on the hair type; in a plastic bowl, place 1-2 full cups of Nupur henna powder. Place one cup of aloe vera juice or coconut milk to one cup of henna mixture or one and half cup of aloe vera juice or coconut milk to two cups henna mixture. Place a 1 ½ tbsp of coconut oil in one cup of henna mixture or 2 1/3 of coconut oil to two cups henna mixture. Add a large egg to the mixture.

2 tbsps of honey or agave nectar to 1 cup of henna mixture or 4 table spoons to 2 cups henna mixture.

Finally add one cup of your favorite moisture rinse out conditioner to one cup of henna mixture or two cups to two cups of henna mixture.

Divide your hair into sections to help even distribution, apply to hair sections and wrap with a plastic cap. Leave on for one to three hours or however long you'd like, and then rinse thoroughly with protein free moisture rich conditioner for bouncy and shiny curls then style as you would.

Allow the water from your shower head to rinse the mixture out, less bending, twisting and manipulation of the hair while the mixture is still in will prevent any tangles and knots from forming.

Coconut Oil Base HOT OIL TREATMENT

I just started using this hot oil treatment for my hair!

Ingredients:

(The amount of ingredients you use depends on the length and thickness of your hair! This is for short-medium length haired people)

1 tablespoons of Castor Oil

2 tablespoons of Coconut Oil

1 tablespoon of Jojoba Oil

2 drops of Vitamin E Oil

1 teaspoon of Peppermint Oil

Olive oil, optional

Directions:

Wash your hair and divide the hair into three to four sections. After your hair has been washed, combine the oils together in a jar or bowl and heat until it is warm and melted (You can heat the oils by placing the jar or bowl in boiled water, or put in a microwave for thirty to forty five seconds). Apply to your scalp and then saturate each section individually.

Keep your plastic cap on for ten to fifteen minutes or sit under a heated dryer or hood for five to ten mins. Finally condition your hair

Pumpkin Seed Butter Mask

This butter mask has a lot of healthy benefits that most people with curls and coils desire and are always trying to incorporate into their hair regimens. This butter mask will promote curl definition and growth.

Ingredients:

2 tablespoons of Sunny Isle Jamaican Black Castor Oil Extra Dark

2 tablespoons of Dastony 100% Organic Sprouted Pumpkin Seed Butter

2 tablespoons of GPB Glycogen Protein Balancing Conditioner

Directions:

Combine equal parts of the Castor Oil, Pumpkin Seed butter and Conditioner. Apply to slightly damp or dry hair. You may need to add more conditioner for easier application on your hair...this mixture does NOT provide slip for your hair, it is a mask, so it just needs to get worked into your hair and on the strands. Wear a plastic shower cap/ plastic bag on it for a minimum of one hour. The mask will become dry stiff. Rinse and cleanse or cowash. You can use it as a pre treatment to your wash day regimen, but you can also use as a deep conditioner as well! (You should still rinse out with a favorite conditioner if you use as a dc, for detangling and to make sure the whole product has been well removed)

Natural hair growth serum

This natural hair growth serum combines essential oils and herbs that are good for hair growth and scalp health:

Nettle: the nettle is rich in vitamins A, vitamin C, vitamin K, Iron, plus magnesium and potassium. It is often used in making natural hair products and it also helps stimulate hair growth.

Horsetail: the horsetail is high in silica and excellent for the hair, as it supports hair growth.

Aloe Vera Gel: the aloevera gel naturally soothes and thickens the scalp and serves as a silkening base for this serum.

Essential Oils: Essential oils of Rosemary, Clary Sage and Lavender are great for hair and scalp health.

Where to Get Ingredients

You can get the horsetail leaf and nettle leaf from Mountain Rose Herbs and the natural aloe vera.

For the essential oils, any high quality option will work. You can order your oils from Mountain Rose Herbs, and Plant Therapy.

Ingredients

1 cup of distilled water

10 drops of Lavender Essential Oil

2 tbsps of Dried Nettle Leaf

10 drops of Rosemary Essential Oil

2 tbsps of Natural Aloe Vera Gel

10 drops of Clary Sage Essential Oil

2 tbsps of Horsetail Leaf (if desired)

Directions:

Boil the distilled water and add the horsetail leaf and dried nettle leaf. Let the herbs sit in the water for a minimum of ten mins or until the water becomes cool. Strain the herbs out and pour the herb infused liquid in to a spray bottle. Add essential oils and the aloe vera and then shake well. Store in the refrigerator for up to three months and shake well before you use.

Spray freely and generously on your hair roots once or more per day. I have found that it was easiest and worked the best to spray on before bed each night.

END

Thank you for reading my book. If you enjoyed it, won't you please take a moment to look at my other titles?

Thanks!

Nancy Crews